Gracefully Diminished: Living with a Traumatic Brain Injury

Mike Kerrey

Published by Mike Kerrey, 2022.

GRACEFULLY DIMINISHED: LIVING WITH A TRAUMATIC BRAIN INJURY

First edition. June 23, 2022.

ISBN: 979-8201540319

Written by Mike Kerrey.

Table of Contents

PART ONE – Introduction

Here we go...hope this helps someone.

Why this book

A doctor first talked to me about having a Traumatic Brain Injury (TBI) about a year after a bus ran into me.

My first response was "What the heck is a TBI?"

I knew nothing about TBIs.

I searched bookstores, the Internet and asked doctors but found few usable resources on Traumatic Brain Injuries. Most of the articles on the Internet were way too technical. For many you had to subscribe to medical sites. There weren't many materials that I could understand or relate to.

I kept wishing for a little book of how people successfully dealt with their TBIs. I could only find a couple sources and hungered for more. So I decided to write down what I had experienced and learned after living with a TBI for eight years. Hopefully it will help someone achieve Peace a little bit quicker, or help a friend or family member gain some Understanding. Maybe someone will learn they aren't alone... that others have gone through something similar and found a good outcome.

This book is broken into the following sections:

1) Identifying

2) Understanding

3) Accepting

4) Living Gracefully

5) Examples

GRACEFULLY DIMINISHED: LIVING WITH A TRAUMATIC BRAIN INJURY

I am not a doctor. Over the last eight years I have seen dozens of doctors and therapists. I have been to hundreds of appointments. I have been tested and retested. I have read everything that I could find. I have tried dozens of treatments. I have learned a lot.

These four words are now my mantra: Understand. Accept. Live Gracefully.

Good luck.

Not Alone

Eighteen months after my accident I went to a going away party for an old friend. At the small party I ran into a past co-worker, 'Jane', who had fallen and hit her head. She also had a TBI. We were both in the middle of our therapies.

Jane was a very bright person with a lot of good experience in our industry. I had really enjoyed working with her because of her intelligence, humor and competence.

Talking to her made me feel better in many ways.

After talking with her I no longer felt so alone. We talked for a long time. We were experiencing similar issues. Not just the cognitive and emotional problems but also the same frustrations dealing with doctors and just people in general.

We shared experiences with medications. I took her suggestions back to my doctor. She took the name of my neuropsychologist.

We both had been smart with strong memories and good communication skills. Now we both had sporadic cognitive problems.

People treat you so differently when they find out you have cognitive, memory or emotional problems. Lack of trust. No longer comfortable being around you. Trying to do everything for you.

What a life-changing fall from grace. No longer on top of the world. Lots of struggling, fear and frustration. Failure.

That chance meeting is one of the big reasons I wrote this book. Instead of relying on a chance meeting, maybe someone will be helped by reading about my experiences. Maybe find their own path to Living Gracefully. Or, maybe, just not feel so alone.

Bang

A Traumatic Brain Injury can be caused by a sports injury, a car accident, a fall or basically anything that causes a blow to the head. The injury can range from an open head wound to internal bleeding and bruising or microscopic damage that doesn't show up on any scans. The brain injury can occur by itself or as part of trauma to other areas of the body. The injury can be obvious and life threatening or hidden and difficult to identify.

In April of 2012, I was walking across a street and was struck by a turning shuttle bus. I saw it out of the corner of my vision and had time to throw up my left arm in front of my head. The next thing I remember is picking myself off of the pavement. My left leg wouldn't work and my left hand was stiff. I was bleeding from my back, shoulders and upper arms from road rash. I had been thrown at least ten feet. I was seeing stars. My only thought was to hop out of the street so I wouldn't be run over by another car. Luckily some construction workers hustled over to help me get to the grass. They held me up as I didn't want to try to sit because I thought my left hip was broken. As they held me up, I went in and out of consciousness. When I was awake I was still seeing stars.

In the ambulance, the police officer told me to be happy that my left arm was broken. The cushioning it had provided had probably saved my life.

At the hospital I found out my left knee that was broken (tibia plateau fracture), not my left hip. One of many examples of confusion after an accident. My vision alternated between clear and stars. They immobilized my left arm. Then head/brain/neck scans. Nothing showed on the scans. The focus shifted to my broken bones. And the pain medications started. They waited a day to operate on my knee and wrist to allow the swelling to go down. In addition to the wrist and knee surgeries, they had to do a ten inch 'compartment' incision in my lower leg to reduce the chance of swelling and infection. Hardware (20 pins, plates and screws) was used to put things back in place. More pain medications.

I was released from the hospital after five days and then had a 24-hour, 1,400-mile drive back home while laying across the backseat of a rental car. The pain medications were causing me to hallucinate. About 18 hours into the drive I quit taking the pain medications...didn't like seeing trees trying to attack the car. Walker at rest stops. A brief hotel stop so I could stretch out.

Finally I was home again with a huge sigh of relief.

Who I Was

It took me a while to understand but that instant of getting hit by the shuttle bus made me a different person.

I started to feel like a stranger.

No longer myself. I could be sitting with a group of old friends or family and feel completely out of place. I didn't belong. A stranger among friends. A stranger to myself. Alone. I didn't like that stranger. I quickly came to hate that person. Thought about killing him. Didn't understand him. So different. A complete failure.

No idea who I was.

PART TWO - Identifying

TBIs are difficult to identify and are often identified too late.

Triage

Triage is used by emergency rooms and hospitals to prioritize treatment. The ripples of triage continued to affect me for a year.

In my case, the emergency room doctors focused first on my head because I had hit it, had gone in and out of consciousness and had vision problems. They ran brain/head/neck scans and x-rays. When nothing bad showed on those tests they moved on to the broken bones. At some point they cleaned up the road rash on the back of my arms and shoulders from when I had landed and skidded on the pavement.

Over the next six months my treatment focused on my leg and wrist. It included another surgery on the wrist to remove some of that hardware. Physical therapy three times a week for both leg and arm to strengthen and work on range of movement. Progression from wheel chair to walker to crutch to cane to just walking! Then walking longer and longer distances.

Later, doctors said that many minor and medium Traumatic Brain Injuries are not identified for months or even years after the injury. Often, as in my case, there are other injuries that require all of the person's focus and energy. They are going through recovery and convalescence. Often times they are on significant pain medications that further hide cognitive issues. The injured and their family are in a non-familiar environments and circumstances. Trips to the doctor and physical therapy. Daily activities that we normally taken for granted are now a chore (going to the bathroom, eating, moving, etc.). Just getting through a day exhausts the injured and their family.

So it turns out that the major impact of the bus breaking my leg and arm was not the actual breaks but the fact that they helped mask the

TBI. They delayed the start of my TBI therapy until after the normal nine-to-twelve-month TBI recovery period.

Houston, We Have a Problem

I started to notice that something wasn't right with my head through a gradual process. It was gradual because there were a lot of other 'noise' and activities going on. My friends brought me books and movies. I tried and couldn't read the books or watch movies. I put them aside. I was constantly exhausted and emotional. When I wasn't going to a doctor or therapist or doing at home exercises I sat in a chair, slept or watched TV.

One of the identification difficulties is that when problems happen at home it is very easy to ignore them. Since many of my problems were cognitive, my own diminished thought processes helped hide them. The hospital tests hadn't found anything wrong with my brain so I must be okay. Plus, I wasn't used to identifying and dealing with these types of issues.

And my problems were sporadic and varied:

- Reading was difficult/impossible

- Trouble watching movies

- Problems focusing in restaurants or stores

- Trouble totaling a credit card receipt

- Couldn't recall names (kids, friends and co-workers)

- Couldn't recall basic info (addresses and phone numbers)

When I returned to work my problems became very obvious and impossible to ignore. But I got good at finding excuses to hide my problems:

- Negotiating with a client on a contract and couldn't recall basic terms that I had used hundreds of times before. I broke down in tears and had to excuse myself because 'something was in my eye'.

- After a meeting with the senior management of a very important client, my client asked me if had fallen asleep in the meeting as I didn't respond to any of their questions. To this day I still can't recall any of the meeting. I used 'sorry feel like I have the flu.'

- Flew out and met with a prospective client on Friday. On Monday that person called me and I couldn't recall who he was, the trip or the meeting. I broke off the phone call because 'someone was at the door'. It bought me time to check my airline reservations to find out where I had traveled. Then searched my email for that town so I could find emails from that client and figure out who had called me.

- Went to see a prospective client to discuss a new insurance product. When the meeting started I couldn't recall anything about the product. Stopped the meeting so 'I could use the rest room' and I used the break to look up the product on my phone.

- I froze in a meeting with a room of co-workers. Tears started to run down my face. We had to take a break. Again I used 'something in my eye'.

- In another meeting I couldn't read the words on the white board or do some basic math. Stopped the meeting and went home because 'had the flu'.

These all happened within a span of a couple of weeks. I had to face the fact that I had serious problems. I finally went in to see my doctor. I was immediately referred to a neuropsychologist. It took a couple more months to get an appointment with the neuropsychologist.

I continued to try to work even after I started treatment with my neuropsych. I was working and going through neuropsych sessions, vision therapy, evaluations, coping therapy etc. Problems continued to happen at work. It wasn't getting better. Also doctor appointments were rescheduled or skipped due to work travel. Finally I had to decide to take a leave of absence from work to focus on my medical issues. I didn't want my reputation to suffer or to hurt my company's reputation.

My problems could have been significantly worse. I could have been dead. Or non-functioning. Or in wheel chair. Or not able to talk. Or not able to control my limbs. Much, much worse. However, one of the biggest issues with a minor/medium TBI is that it is not obvious. Not obvious for initial identification. Not obvious to yourself. Not obvious to others. Friends and co-workers thought I was goofing around when I couldn't remember basic things. Or hit a golf ball. Or read a menu. Or talk about the football game from yesterday.

It isn't easy to accept that you might have cognitive issues. I wish I would have paid more attention to the early signs. I wish I would have gone to a doctor quicker. By the time I first saw a neuropsychologist it was between six to nine months after the accident...well through most of the natural recovery plateaus of the brain. The identification and treatment process takes time. By the time I got appointments to see some of the specialists it was well over eighteen months after the accident. Many of the doctors would just shrug after they heard the amount of time that had elapsed. They knew that most TBI improvements happened in the first twelve months after the injury. I started to hear 'permanent after this amount of time' and 'chronic'.

Speed of identification is key to aiding recovery. If in doubt go see your doctor. Make it a priority. It is important.

Agreement

Treatment is full of frustrations. One of the biggest is that the doctors don't always agree. There are a tremendous amount of unknowns when it comes to Traumatic Brain Injuries.

Here are the items that most of the doctors agreed upon:

- A TBI often does not show up on brain scans.

- Identification of a TBI is often delayed.

- The human brain repairs itself through a series of plateaus over the first nine to twelve months after the injury.

- After twelve months, a TBI is unlikely to get better. It is chronic. It is forever.

- A TBI spawns many problems.

- Now for some good news: A TBI is NOT degenerative. It does not get worse over time. And the problems it spawns also do not get worse over the years.

The only way the problems get worse over time is if a person's responses to the problems gets worse. If you don't deal with them then you can get into a downward spiral emotionally and socially. And that downward spiral can accelerate. It is important to figure out how to respond to the problems. That is in your control.

Knowledge

Knowledge was the most important thing I gained from over a hundred visits to doctors and therapists for my TBI. Like most people, I had heard of Traumatic Brain Injury because it was a hot topic in the news. TBIs were mainly caused by sport injuries from playing football or soccer and were significant problems with our military due to explosions.

It was never something that I had ever expected to deal with.

Luckily my neuropsychologist (Dr A) helped me. He saved my life both literally and qualitatively. We meshed. Maybe he was too blunt for other patients but I wanted the truth and didn't need it sugar coated. Also, we are both golf fanatics so it gave us something in common. And we are both very strong family men. Anyway...that meshing was important to me then and is still to this day. I knew he cared.

All of the doctors and therapists discussed how TBIs introduced problems that I had to deal with but it was my neuropsych that formed the foundation of my learning and eventual success. Dr A created a path to Living Gracefully. There were three main steps that he showed me:

Understanding

Accepting

Living Gracefully

The next three sections go into these topics and how they are key to achieving happiness.

PART THREE - Understanding

The first step to achieving a graceful life is to Understand.

Chronic

Chronic means forever.

A doctor would say my TBI is chronic. My response would be, "OK. How do we fix it?" The doctor would respond it is permanent. And I would say, "OK. But what is the treatment?"

Other doctors would say, "A really long time", or "No chance". Often I thought they were just trying manage my expectations and that there was a cure. They had to say it dozens of times in different ways before it began to sink in.

After a life as a problem solver, I was being told there was no fix to my biggest problem.

They were all saying the same thing. I had reached a point where my TBI was forever.

Inventory

Several doctors said to keep lists and logs. Logs provide information and perspective on your problems. You can spot trends. They help you understand your problems. Frequency. Intensity. Activities that Trigger problems. Activities that mitigate problems.

One of the basic logs is a headache log. For months, I kept a little notebook in my pocket. Every hour I logged the intensity and location of my headaches. I used a scale of 1 to 10 which is what most doctors wanted. It was very eye-opening. Most days I woke up with a low headache. By noon it had increased. By afternoon it was increasing faster. By evening it had maxed out.

And there were logs for cognitive and vision problems.

I started recording my activities each hour alongside my problems. That helped identify Triggers.

Another doctor had me track what I was eating to see if certain foods effected my TBI problems. In my case it wasn't.

When you are in pain you don't think clearly. Also, while experiencing a cognitive problem isn't the best time to solve problems. By having it written down, I could review it when I was thinking better.

Data shifts from impression, guessing and opinions to facts and trends. It is impersonal.

The logs helped us to Understand.

Unpredictable, Triggers and Compounding

One of the most frustrating aspects of TBI problems is their unpredictability.

Sometimes the whole sequence happens in minutes. Other times hours.

Several trends emerged from the logs:

1) Sometimes we could see reoccurring patterns before a problem occurred or before it ramped up quickly. A doctor referred to these as 'Triggers'. They encouraged me to make a list of these Triggers. Then we worked on ways to avoid or cope with the Triggers.

2) When I was already experiencing a problem and a different problem occurred the first problem would escalate rapidly. Not only that, but it seemed as if a third problem was likely to happen. One of my doctors described this as similar to the power of compound interest. We called the effect of multiple problems ramping up on top of each other as 'Compounding'. In these cases 1+1 did not equal 2. Sometimes 1+1 equaled 3 or 4 or more.

3) The problems normally get worse as the day goes on. I get very tired both emotionally and physically. And being tired is a Trigger. A bad cycle.

4) Underlying all of this was the unpredictability of the TBI problems. I can be going along and doing fine. Then something starts to go wrong. Maybe it is my vision and I start seeing double. Then my head starts to hurt by my

left temple. And then it gets worse. Then the back of my head starts to hurt. Although we identified some Triggers the problems would sometimes happen independently of any known Trigger.

So..largely unpredictable. Triggers can cause problems. Problems can also occur without a known Trigger. Multiple problems lead to escalation of the intensity of the problems through Compounding. And things get worse as the day goes on. The problems leave me emotionally and physically exhausted.

Even with increased understanding of the Triggers, the problems from the TBI are still largely unpredictable.

I constantly try to figure out patterns and more Triggers.

Sometimes I can predict how I am going to feel. Sometimes I can understand how I got to lying on the basement floor in a ball. The majority of the time I can't. It doesn't follow a known pattern. Some days I just wake up seeing double with a bad headache. Already tired and the day hasn't started. My response now is to get on the treadmill and start walking. And walk till I feel better or my knee or hip can't do any more. Try to power past the problems. Just Shake My Head and keep going.

I can be in a quiet room talking with a friend feeling good. All of a sudden I can't recall the person's name. Or what we were talking about. Or what is he doing in our house. Or the address of our house.

Unpredictable.

As problem solvers and programmers, my wife and I struggled with it being unpredictable. There should be logical reasons. We constantly tried to debug. I had to stop trying to debug the TBI. It isn't a computer program. It is a Traumatic Brain Injury. It is mostly unpredictable.

Understand. Accept.

Blackness

A little bit on memory:

Memory is composed of three main activities:

- Putting into memory

- Storing memories

- Recalling memories

As things are put into memory they include different indexes that relate to that item. A single item can have many indexes. For example, your first car can be indexed by model, make, color, driving it for the first time, new car smell, feel of the upholstery, getting a ticket, a vacation, a date, a fender bender, the license plate number or making car payments. There can be hundreds of these indexes for a single item.

Also memory is often divided into short term (recent happenings) and long term (older things).

Memory problems can happen with any of these activities. They can be focused on just short term or long term or both.

My Problem:

My problems are recall problems...getting something from memory. This recall problem is for both short and long term. My indexing works fine. The problem occurs just at the last instant of recalling something. Instead of getting my daughter's name I fall into Blackness. Or instead of recalling that 3 times 6 is 18 I get Blackness.

This memory recall failure differs from normal 'just not remembering something' or 'tip of the tongue' or just plain not knowing something.

It is distinct. There is this feeling of complete wrongness. And falling. And Blackness.

When I can't recall something it feels like I am falling into a never-ending Blackness. It includes all the emotions you get with falling...fear, panic, out of control, etc. But unlike a regular fall this Blackness goes on and on. Sometimes I get locked into it and it can last seconds or minutes. Falling into Blackness.

One pattern is that once a problem occurs recalling an item, I will likely have problems again and again recalling that same item. With math it is recalling addition, subtraction, multiplication and division tables for 3s and 7s. I never have problems with other numbers. Trying to use a 3 or 7 sometimes recalls blackness instead of the correct answer.

I went to many sessions on memory therapy to learn recall techniques. Most of the techniques didn't work. Some are very basic. For example, if you can't recall your first car by using model then use the color. And if color doesn't work then use a smell or texture. Or an event with the car. Once I got Blackness, using other indexes also recalled Blackness. Then maybe they work with no problem an hour or a day later.

The main thing I learned from those therapy sessions was to focus on controlling how I reacted to the falling and Blackness. Understand what is happening. Reduce panic. Reduce fear. Don't be embarrassed. This was a huge benefit. It reduced how long I locked up when the recall problem happened. I don't stammer as much or sit in silence as long. Less tears.

The more I Understand a problem the more I can Accept and then avoid or cope with it.

Recall

As mentioned earlier the main takeaway from all of my therapy sessions was an increased Understanding of Traumatic Brain Injuries and my problems.

One of the huge gains was Understanding that my 'memory' problems were mainly recall problems – getting information out of the brain.

During a vision therapy session, I was supposed to read the letters off of an eye chart. I was failing on certain letters. Couldn't recall the name of the letter. When we used a chart that was just arrows – left, right, up and down, I couldn't point in the direction of the arrows. Very frustrating. We took a break then came back to the letter chart. I started rattling off all of the letters. Then the doctor noticed my eyes were shut! I was doing it solely from memory. He had me do it again. No problem while my eyes were shut. Opened my eyes and I couldn't do it. Opened my eyes and faced a blank wall and I could recite the letters. Huge breakthrough. It showed that getting information into my brain and storing it was working ok. My problem was recalling it. And my problem was much more intense and frequent when having sensory input.

Understanding this made a huge difference to me. I wasn't stupid, I just couldn't get the info out. Hadn't forgotten everything. In fact, probably hadn't forgotten any more than a normal person. Just had recall problems at times. Unpredictable...yes. Frustrating...yes. Hopeless...no.

So...I often work on the computer in the dark. Not because the light bothers me but to reduce what I see. Similarly I like it dark to watch TV or a movie. When I start to have problems, I take a break. Shut my eyes. Go to a quiet room. Focus on a single item. Find ways to minimize sensory overload.

Now take the eye chart experience and compare it to reading a book. A single page in a book typically has about 250 words. Lots of sensory input. Also, a lot of recall is needed as a person reads to put the current word or sentence in context with the words before it. Prior sentences. Prior paragraphs. Prior chapters. Or a prior book in a series. Or prior experiences, such as from school twenty years earlier. Reading is surprisingly interactive – new material requires constant recall of memories to make sense of the new words. Reading is a pain for me.

Understand. Accept. Live Gracefully.

Headaches

My headaches start in my left temple. As they get more intense the lower back of my head will start to hurt. And then both areas get more and more painful. When they are really bad, my neck and shoulders get very, very tense.

The headaches can be Triggered by many things or just start for no known reason.

Some days I just wake up with a headache. When I wake up and feel the pain, I don't want to get up but the worse thing I can do is just lay there and worry about it. The best thing is to hop up and start exercising or go take a hot shower.

If I had a really bad day of intense headaches I can wake up after a full night's sleep feeling hungover and exhausted. My body just feels tired. It always seems unfair to wake up hungover without having the fun of a party!

I often go to bed with a bad headache.

These headaches are not like migraines except in the intensity. I had migraines before but haven't for 10+ years. Several doctors tested me to see if these are normal migraines (triggers such as flashing lights). They aren't.

A headache-free hour is rare. A headache-free day is almost unknown. Celebrate pain-free moments.

Vision

Vision problems might be my goofiest problems. Thanks to scores of visits to two different vision specialists I have gained Understanding and insight. Nothing is fixed. But I understand what is happening. I have identified some Triggers. And some coping activities.

When I am focused on an item and something else moves my brain 'sees' the first item move. Never sure when this will happen. Trying to read a road sign. It can start to move. Focused on my golf ball and the club starts the backswing then the ball moves. Really weird stuff. It only happens when I focus on something so no problems accurately seeing other cars, etc. If I shut my left eye the problem goes away. If I open my left eye the problem can start up again.

Often I will see double on items within a couple feet of me. Icons on the computer screen. Words on a page. Water glasses at the table. Two golf balls. It can be anything. Again, closing my left eye helps. The eye doctor and therapists also taught me several techniques such as focusing on a distant item like the corner of a door and then moving my focus from corner to corner of the door. Or I put items on the floor under a table and use those to focus on. Or sticking out my thumb and focusing on it while I move it closer and then away from me (called tromboning).

Or sometimes it is the frustrating search for an item that is right in front of me and never seeing it. Maybe a book on a shelf. Or a type of cereal in the store. Or a specific shirt hanging on a rack of shirts. Or an item on a menu. Sometimes closing my left eye helps. Other times I just have to walk away and try later.

As you can imagine reading is highly problematic when the vision problems are acting up.

Basically, the brain injury broke how my brain coordinates and combines signals from both eyes. Also, now my right eye is extremely dominant over my left. The two eyes don't work together any more (teaming).

I also now have a centerline shift which means the center of my vision is not in the correct alignment. Instead of being in the true center my center is shifted to the right.

Often I will discover that my left eye is partially or fully shut without me intentionally shutting it. My body has learned how to cope with some of these problems.

When my left eye shuts down my head will shift more to the left to align my vision to the center. This puts more strain on my neck being in an unnatural position for long time periods.

Goofy!

At least we identified and gained some Understanding of the problems. Not as scared now when problems happen. Take them in stride and just move on.

Not Problems

It is also important to understand what are not Triggers. I didn't pay enough attention to this in the beginning. I was tested a lot and only focused on the Triggers. Should also have kept a list of the items that were not Triggers for me.

Smell

Sounds

Touch

Light (bright, strobing, different colors, intensity)

Food

Relief

Just as certain things act as Triggers there are activities that seem to mitigate those Triggers. Not a fix. Just makes it better.

Hot, hot showers

Exercise

Being outside

Empty walls

Hot tubs

Caveat

One huge caveat about Understanding – some things just have to be Accepted as not understandable. No reason. No logic.

Don't struggle too much. Understand that some things are just not understandable. Just Accept. And move on.

Can't find peace if you constantly struggle to find logic and to understand.

Some things about a TBI and the resulting problems just don't make sense. No rhyme or reason.

The end goal is Peace and Happiness. Anything that gets in the way or slows up the process needs to be looked at hard. Is it needed? Can it be changed? Can it be dropped? Replaced?

So sometimes it is Understanding that you won't fully Understand. And Accepting.

Medications

Dozens of medications produced mixed and limited results. And the intent of these medications was to address the symptoms of the TBI...not to fix it.

Most of the prescriptions for my headaches started at a low dose and increased over weeks. The same process but in reverse is required to get off of that medication. Be sure to talk to your doctor and follow the directions exactly. None of these medications provided any noticeable relief. My doctors said that is not unusual.

Also be aware that these medications are potent and not without side effects:

- One of the medications triggered a ringing in my right ear. Even after working my way off of the medication the ringing continues. The ringing has continued for almost a year now. My doctor researched the medication and said the medication triggers permanent ear ringing in about four percent of people taking it. Would rather have won the Powerball.

- Another medication caused my face, hands and feet to go numb. The numbness left my hands and feet a couple of days after stopping that medication. My face took about ten days to completely lose the numbness.

My friend who also had a TBI suggested a muscle relaxant to help with the headaches and tense neck and shoulders. When I took that suggestion to my doctor he agreed and prescribed one. It helped. At first I used it daily. Now after making progress on finding other techniques to mitigate the pain (exercising, walking, taking breaks, etc.) I only use the muscle relaxant in extreme cases.

Regular headache medicines like aspirin and Tylenol did not help.

I have tried many supplements. No bad effects. Maybe some good help. Again, some of these are supposed to be much more helpful when used soon after the injury. They reportedly help the brain help itself repair. Unfortunately, I didn't try any of these until more than 24 months after the injury.

My main learning on this was to see your doctor early and often. Be completely open. Don't minimize your problems. Find doctors you are comfortable with and trust, then work diligently for solutions. Keep trying.

Work

Work was a cornerstone of my life. It was a huge piece of how I defined myself.

And I was lucky – I loved my job. For over twenty-five years I had learned and grown within the same industry. We designed computer systems, built processes and teams of people that serviced insurance policies. In one year, we handled transactions that exceeded seven billion dollars. Our company had about twenty people working there when I started. When we sold it, we had over 1,300 employees. We rented the local arena for our Christmas parties. It was a blast.

At the end I was traveling over 40 weeks a year helping design insurance products and build the teams to provide the service. Lucky to work with friends that were incredibly fun and terrific at their jobs.

That all came to an end with the TBI. Huge hole in my life. Hundreds of hours a month to fill. Lost a bunch of friends.

I miss working. The challenges. The successes. The people.

Doctors

This is a sad subject. One of the huge disappointments and frustrations of my whole experience.

My prior experiences with doctors had been largely positive. Then my accident happened.

One glaring gap in my treatment was someone to manage the process. Each doctor was focused on a niche. No doctor or therapist oversaw the entire process. Those niches didn't communicate well. They would forward records to the next doctor but only if I asked. And it could take weeks or months to happen. Scheduling and even finding the specialists mostly fell to me. It was exhausting. This whole process fell to the person with the Traumatic Brain Injury.

In my case, since the problems were caused by a shuttle bus hitting me as I walked across the street, there were insurance claims and lawyers involved. I quickly found out that the medical field is hugely influenced by how the injury happened, insurance and possible litigation.

A doctor who I had seen in the past refused to see me when he found out about a possible insurance claim.

Another doctor asked me to come back if a certain condition reoccurred. It did reoccur. I made an appointment to see him. Then his office manager called back to cancel the appointment. The reason was his corporate rules would not allow me to come back since the insurance company had closed the claim. I even offered to pay cash to get his help. Still got turned down because they didn't want to 'violate their insurance company relationship'.

A therapist told me that her organization had decided to become more friendly to insurance companies and had hired a consultant to change their processes.

Doctors are forced to choose sides between patients and insurance companies.

All I wanted was help.

Two doctors stuck by me through the years and stayed focused solely on my well-being. I will always be in their debt.

PART FOUR – Accepting

Acceptance is not easy and took me the longest to achieve.

Acceptance

Several of the doctors talked about me needing to Accept what had happened. I thought this was weird. Of course, I had been hit by a shuttle bus. I knew that. No doubt there. I had been in a wheel chair. I still walked with a limp. It was dramatic. Wasn't likely to forget it.

What they were really saying (and what I was avoiding) was that I had a Traumatic Brain Injury. And at this point it was not going to get any better. Until I Accepted my situation I couldn't make real progress. Every doctor was telling me the same thing. Some couched it with "don't expect" or "we can try". My neuropsych and General Practitioner were the most direct and I appreciated that.

I also needed to Accept that I was never going to get back to the person I was before the Traumatic Brain Injury. I needed to Accept who I was now and move forward. That stranger was me. Understand him. Redefine him. Accept him.

Each problem created by the TBI had to be Understood and Accepted. A long, never-ending process.

It took months for me to understand their message.

Finally I started to Accept.

Hope

One of the first discussions about Acceptance with Dr A centered on Hope. His first point was that when dealing with a chronic issue like a Traumatic Brain Injury is that Hope is Bad. Sounds very harsh. But it is true. We spent hours on this subject.

One of the few things that my doctors were consistent about is that there is No Cure for my TBI. I didn't have bleeding or bruising that could be fixed with surgery. My brain had been bounced when struck by the bus and when I landed on the pavement. The damage was at such a microscopic level that it didn't show on MRI or other scans. That this was normal in the majority of TBI cases! And if you can't find the problem you can't fix it! No miracle pill. No Cure.

The brain itself will attempt repairs. These occur in roughly three-month plateaus for the first nine to twelve months following the injury. Many of the therapists felt that their activities could help the brain repair during these plateaus. That is one reason that early detection of a TBI is critical. But many TBIs are like mine...they are not identified until many months after the injury. In my case it was about nine months since the shuttle bus hit me until I saw a doctor about the TBI.

If you can't fix it then it is chronic. In chronic situations Hope is Bad. Harsh but true.

Why is Hope Bad?

Hope delays moving on to Acceptance and the next stages in the process.

Hope is false. Hope causes you to expend emotional and physical energy on activities that don't move you forward. That energy is in critically short supply.

Hope increases the height and depth of the emotional roller coaster that a TBI creates in your life. Each new doctor or therapy represents a shining new hope. And then, disappointment. Instead, they are better viewed as new opportunities for learning. Paths to Understanding. Avoidance skills. Coping skills. Getting retrained. Redefined. Strive to be emotionally level. No artificial highs. No emotional crashes.

Hope makes it tougher on the people close to you - spouse, kids, friends.

Hope leads to constant failure. Bad thoughts.

Acceptance is impossible to achieve while you are being driven by Hope.

Bad Thoughts

About a year after the accident, thinking about suicide started to happen more and more. Then 'ending it' transitioned to planning out the best way. A shotgun? If so, what type of ammo? And where to do it? Outside might be best so the carpet and paint don't get ruined. If not a gun then driving my car into something. Maybe take out more life insurance and make it look like an accident so my family could benefit. Amazing how many ways there are to die. Not good thoughts. Bad Thoughts.

I started to keep notes about thinking about suicide. A trend developed from the notes. Those Bad Thoughts were being driven by extreme feelings of worthlessness and failure. Something would happen and then my thoughts would spiral down and down.

Maybe it was something as simple as adding some numbers like 3+4 when helping a grandson with math. Instead of being able to recall the answer I would fall into Blackness. Failure. I am fifty years old and can't add 3 and 4. Failure. My six-year-old grandson can do that but I can't. Failure. I won the National Math contest in high school and I can't do addition now. Failure. From failure it was an easy transition to worthless. I can't help my grandson. Worthless. I can't pay the bills. Worthless. I can't work and earn money. Worthless. I can't add the credit card receipt. Worthless. An extreme embarrassment. No value. No reason to live. A bad spiral.

Bad Thoughts.

Hope accelerates the Bad Thoughts.

A new treatment naturally would trigger new Hope of a cure. I can be fixed. An emotional high. Ten visits later with lots of expended physical and emotional energy, no improvement. Failure again. The doctors would start out so positive then come back and say no real improvement. Chronic. Hope was shattered. Fall from the emotional high. Failure. Other patients must be able to succeed but I failed. I can't even do this right. Failure. Downward spiral. Bad Thoughts.

This went on for about 18 months. I hadn't ever had to deal with Bad Thoughts before. This was all new to me.

I didn't try to deal with the Bad Thoughts by myself. When the downward spiral got too bad I would talk with my doctors. Or my lead lawyer. I found ways to stop the spirals.

The speed of the downward spirals was increased by failed Hope. Hope was a false high. A bad drug. Lots of highs followed by lower lows. A crutch. Hope stopped me from Accepting my situation and just dealing with it. Just one more doctor and things will get better. The next medication will fix my headaches. The next glasses will let me read. Hope and failure. Not a good combination. Hope created a lot of Bad Thoughts.

Bad Thoughts were new to me. I had to map out a plan to avoid them.

Understanding. Acceptance. Living Gracefully.

Peace

Of all of the concepts I have heard over the last eight years, oddly enough, Peace was the hardest for me to grasp. Peace is foundational for Happiness. Dr A and several of the doctors kept coming back to Peace.

I had to redefine myself to achieve peace. Constant feelings of failure destroy peace.

Peace is only achieved through Acceptance. I had to Accept that I had a chronic injury. Stop Hoping. Start Accepting and moving on. The problems were forever. For me Acceptance was only possible after Understanding.

No big ah-ha moment. Just worked on each problem. Gain some Understanding. Move to Acceptance. Gain more Peace.

A highly iterative process. Treat everything as small problems. Celebrate each little gain. Go for incremental improvements. Never ending. Still surprised every day by new twists on problems. Not failure. Many small successes.

Understand. Accept. Living Gracefully.

PART FIVE - Living Gracefully

The goal for the rest of my life.

Gracefully Diminished

The harshest words in my life were when my neuropsychologist, Dr A, said my new goal in life was to be 'Gracefully Diminished'. Wow. Pretty hard hitting. But as soon as he said those words, I understood them. And Accepted them. Everything suddenly clicked. It was a turning point.

Diminished?

Graceful?

That night I didn't sleep as I thought of those two words.

Huge impact.

What did I need to do to live Gracefully Diminished?

Huge challenge. There are so many levels of meaning to those words.

Yes, I was Diminished.

Very different person than I had been before the accident. My skills and abilities were less. Not bad. Just less. Less in many ways. Better off than many. Still smart. Still a good person. Physically strong. Lots of support. Great family. Great friends.

We started working on redefining how I thought of myself. Get rid of that stranger. Understand myself. Create a definition where I could be a success. Define my goals so I could win and not view myself as a constant failure.

De-emphasize the diminished skills. Accept them. Build on the strengths.

Was I Graceful? No. Not yet.

I was full of anger, frustration, feelings of failure, thoughts of suicide and hate. I hated myself because I was failing every hour, every day. Redefine. Keep what was important and achievable. Change my priorities. Get rid of hate. Stop the Bad Thoughts. Shift focus to values. Family. Friends. Experiences.

To achieve Graceful I had to become at Peace with the new me. Strike a good balance. Use Understanding and Acceptance to become Peaceful. Peace. Graceful.

I often look to the Serenity Prayer. There aren't many words but it is very powerful.

Give us the serenity to accept what cannot be changed,

The courage to change what can be changed,

and the wisdom to know one from the other.

I'm not a religious person but I constantly go back to these three lines. Some versions of it actually include 'Grace': 'Give me Grace to accept with serenity'.

The three steps Dr A outlined map very closely to the Serenity Prayer.

Serenity is Peace.

An important point: Gracefully Diminished does not mean giving up. In fact, it includes never giving up.

Know what can be changed. Work to change those items. Keep trying new ways to address problems: medications, trigger point therapy, massage, exercise, chiropractor visits, etc. In fact my definition of Graceful includes never giving up. Do the most I can. The courage to change what can be changed.

It helped greatly to view all problems as small. If it seems huge then break it into pieces. Manageable pieces. Don't sweat the small things. Break big hills into small steps.

The Understanding to know what can be changed and what can't. Focus your limited energy on what can be changed.

Back in junior high, we had to read Ernest Hemingway's The Old Man and the Sea. It seemed to me at the time that the book and the teacher droned on and on. She kept talking about how the Old Man was Graceful. Graceful in the face of challenges. He never gave up. He fought the big fish. He fought the sea. He fought the sharks. He fought. And fought. He dealt with one bad situation after another. Went from having a huge fish to just the skeleton left. Never gave up. Graceful. If I ever meet Mrs. Larson again I will thank her for teaching me that lesson. After Dr A said my goal was to be successfully Gracefully Diminished, the Old Man and his struggle came back to me. Be Graceful. Never give up. Keep moving forward.

Now after years of work, people often can't tell when I am experiencing problems. Success. The bad problems are still noticeable but the lower level, high frequency problems don't show as much. Success. The problems don't stop me. Success.

In all of this, there might appear to be one conflict and that is around Hope. Not for me. I still view Hope as bad. I work to improve the changeable things and never give up but I do it without Hope. No expectation of a miraculous fix. No roller coaster of emotions accelerated up by Hope and dashed down by Hope. No outside force is going to wave a wand. Just me and the fish. And the sharks. And the sea.

Grace and serenity to accept what cannot be changed.

Courage to change what can be changed.

Wisdom to know the one from the other.

Understanding. Accepting. Living Gracefully.

Build a foundation of Acceptance and Peace.

Actively Replace

Life is full of things. It is important to control what fills up your life. Those things influence happiness, depression, etc.

I learned this the hard way. As things dropped out of my life it created a vacuum. Into that vacuum rushed Bad Thoughts. I was failing because I couldn't do the old things. Failure. Withdrawal. Emptiness. Bad Thoughts.

Being busy leaves less time for self-pity or to think about pain.

I have taken up fishing. It takes a lot of time, is outdoors and doesn't trigger many of my problems. Golf is similar. Practice. Hit balls. Or I take a walk, even in the rain. Enjoy being outside. Enjoy the doing.

Find activities to do. Better to do something than sit. Especially sit and wish about old things.

Activities that used to be non-events can now be opportunities to feel successful. Take time doing them. Instead of being an item on a to-do list make it fun and fill time. When going to the grocery store stop and look at something you haven't tried. Instead of just running in and out to get a gallon of milk take the time to walk every aisle. Try the samples. Look at the new items. Enjoy the success. Smell the roses.

Take joy in the small things. The fifteen- or thirty-minute activities.

Replace big activities with small things. Take a walk. Look at old picture albums. Walk through a library. Stop at a park. Look at movie reviews. Plan a trip even if you aren't going. Try out new golf clubs. Walk a sporting goods store. Research a historical event or location. Sit in a mall and watch people. Look for a dream car. Drive past your childhood home.

When I pick up my grandson, I leave plenty early so if I have problems recalling the school or route I have time to recover. Often I am there twenty or thirty minutes early. The old me would have read a book. Now I do things. Good amount of time for a walk around the school or neighborhood. Or time to research something. Or to walk through a nearby store or library. Time to message a friend.

Fill your time with successes. Even small successes. Small successes mean more success.

Redefine

You have to become at Peace with yourself and your situation.

Accept that the Old you is in the past.

Redefine the New you for success and happiness.

If you constantly try for something you are not capable of doing then you are setting yourself up for failure.

Don't be complacent. Constantly redefine yourself to push.

Success. Redefine. Success. Redefine.

Much better than failure and bad thoughts.

Redefine who you are and what is important in your life.

Old Me:

Reader

Valued salary

Loved working and making business deals

Liked being one of the smartest people in the room

Played trivia

Traveled for work most weeks

Good Person

New Me:

Good Person

MIKE KERREY

Husband, Father and Grandfather

Friend

Exerciser

The experience of golfing rather than focusing on the score.

The experience of life without keeping score.

Helping grandkids.

Don't have to know the answer myself just guide them to find their own answer.

Focus more on the journey than on acquiring stuff.

The sound of the surf. The feel of the sand. The heat of the sun.

The good tired of exercising. The sights of a walk.

Fish instead of read.

Don't hope. Actively push to do more.

Slow constant improvements. Peace. Stay off of the emotional roller coaster.

Only you can define yourself.

Too Much Time on My Hands

It seemed liked all of the changes left me with oodles of time. Empty time.

I had to quit working. Bam. An empty eight to ten hours a day.

I had to quit reading. Bam. An empty ten or more hours a week.

No more work travel. Bam. Another empty ten hours a week.

Bam.

Bam.

Boredom.

Lots of time for Bad Thoughts. Lots of time for downward spirals.

Had to redefine to fill up that time with good activities. Success rather than failure.

Walking.

Exercising.

Writing.

Grandkids.

Vacation Travel. Planning travel even if you never go.

Golf.

Fishing.

Fill it up. With success. With happiness.

Asking Is Strength

I used to tell people at work a thousand times that asking for help is a sign of strength. Now I have to live that way. It is difficult.

If I don't ask I often fail.

The biggest problem with asking for help is not the "Are you kidding?" odd look or questions. The biggest risk is that a relationship will change over time. Asking a stranger is easier than asking a family member or a close friend. Less to lose with a stranger.

With friends and family the risk isn't that they will mock me. The risk is that they will try to do more for me. I am already diminished by the TBI so don't diminish me more by taking more away from me. It happens. It is insidious. To a certain degree it is to be expected.

Doesn't mean I have to like it!

Ask when needed. Stay safe. Don't put yourself or others in danger because you are too proud or scared to ask for help. Or, just take a break. Have the wisdom to Understand what you can do safely and when you need help. But don't abdicate. Do what you can do. Have the courage to ask for help.

Who I Am

So after four years I am very different from the person I was prior to the accident and from the stranger.

I have gained understanding of my problems.

I have accepted and moved away from Bad Thoughts.

I have redefined myself and replaced my goals and activities.

Diminished, yes, but also Gracefully Diminished.

PART SIX – Examples

Lessons learned and coping skills.

Problems – Avoiding and Coping

These examples of problems caused by my Traumatic Brain Injury are here to give an idea of how much a person's life can be permanently changed. Also, how weird the problems can be. For most problems there is a way to cope. They can't be fixed or prevented, but you can find a way to cope. No matter how stupid. Or significant. Or insignificant.

Some of these are just laughable they are so weird.

Don't rely on Hope; instead, make small improvements. Incremental improvements add up over time.

Now, most of the time, people can't even tell I have a TBI. Success!

A couple friends asked how I was cured. Wow what a great feeling that was. When I talk to people about the multi-year process they often don't understand. They only view things as either fixed or broken. A binary view on life. The same view I had before the accident.

Life is not black and white but grays. Take the absolutes where the results were likely failures and redefine them to increase your chance of success.

Understand. Accept. Live Gracefully.

Recall

Problem:

Addition/subtraction

Books

Names

Places

Days

Cope:

I can't fix the recall problem but I can improve how I react. I understand and accept the problem. I can recognize the falling into Blackness and not panic

The better I react the quicker I recover from the problem. Most times now people won't see me pause. I might stammer or go quiet but I don't lock up.

Since sensory overload (especially visual) is a key trigger for me, if I start to have problems with recall while talking I often close my eyes, look down, etc.

I prefer areas that aren't busy (lots of people, lots of stuff on the walls, noise, etc.).

Phone Numbers

Problem:

The old me used to remember all kinds of facts - phone numbers, addresses, email address, dates, program names, company names, names of people etc.

Now I am lucky to be able to recall my own phone number.

Even something as simple as trying to write down information like a phone number can be difficult. People just rattle off the ten digits...maybe with two pauses to break it into three groups. It is highly unlikely that I can write fast enough to get all of the numbers written down. My recall just doesn't work well enough.

Cope:

I have gotten really good at saving numbers and info into my phone. If someone offers me their info I ask them to text or email me instead so I can just save the info as a new contact and don't have to try to enter it as they say it.

Or I just hand them a piece of paper and ask them to write down their info instead of telling me and me trying to write it down.

Most of the time I can make my request sound so natural that they don't know I am doing it to avoid my problems.

Forgetting Names

Problem:

Remembering people's names or just problems with names in general.

I often have problems remembering people's names. I know who they are. It was a big stumbling block. I would start out a conversation by greeting them by name and get stuck immediately. Just Blackness.

The names of towns, movies, actors, friends, games, athletes, books, characters, etc.

Avoid/Cope:

Retrained myself to not attempt to say 'Hi Mark." I avoid using their name when I greet someone. Now I just say 'Hi." Might not be as friendly but it helps reduce the odds of me having problems.

As I have slowed my speech I have attempted to build in time so I can silently rehearse the name I am going to say. If I have a recall problem with the name I avoid using it. For example, one of my reoccurring problems is with 'Newport Beach'. We have stayed there frequently and love the area. Almost every time I try to recall it I get Blackness. So now I just default to saying 'the Marriott by our oldest daughter'.

I am retraining myself to use general descriptions and move to specific if I can rehearse the name. For example, I will say our 'winter vacation' instead of 'Manasota Key'.

That Dang I

Problem:

A recent memory recall problem is how to spell my first name. Spelling either Michael or Mike can now Trigger a Recall problem.

I fall into Blackness after the 'M' when I try to recall the 'I'.

Sounds stupid.

This problem followed my typical recall problem pattern.

Something that I knew very well and had recalled hundreds or thousands of times suddenly returned Blackness instead of the correct information.

I had to recover from the Blackness.

There was shock and shame at not being able to spell my first name.

When I tried later (sometimes days later) I could recall it correctly.

And the recall problem now reoccurs sporadically when I try to recall that item (in this case how to spell my first name).

Cope:

Now that I know this is a reoccurring potential recall problem I anticipate the Blackness, take a deep breath and be ready to be at Peace if the problem occurs.

If possible, I delay signing the birthday card or completing the form until I am having minimal problems, or until I am by myself so others can't see me and I don't feel pressure or rushed. If I can't pick the timing then I just move forward.

Also after 50 years I am working to change how I scrawl my signature.

Now instead of writing my first name I am using just my initial - M instead of Mike or Michael.

Passwords

Problem:

Passwords and user ids are everywhere. Every day I use dozens of websites or programs that require the user to login. With my recall problems, I get locked out of some program almost every day. A constant stream of failures.

Cope:

My decades in IT had taught me how important good password management is and to never write down the information.

I had to accept that I couldn't live by those old rules. My recall problems just didn't allow it.

I had to write down and hide the information.

Maybe not the most secure way to handle technology but the best way I could figure out how to do it and to be successful.

Take the Long Way Home

Problem:

When driving somewhere I can't recall how to get there. I can't recall the route or the street names or street grid.

I have lived in my home town over 40 years and know it very well. I have lived in the same general area for 20 of those years. The town is laid out in a simple grid. Easy to get around. Except when I can't recall how to get somewhere!

Cope:

With today's technology there is a simple way to deal with this - always use the GPS in my car. I have refused to do that. Driving is very important to me. I don't want to give up any part of it. It is freedom. Turning even a part of that freedom over to a computer seems like failure to me. Don't want instructions constantly in my life. It is important to retain what is important.

I have always been early. Now I leave even earlier so when I have recall problems I can still be on time.

When traveling cross country I normally use the GPS just like a person without recall problems would do. It's just the smart thing to do.

In my hometown, when I have problems recalling the route and am pressed for time or the driving conditions are poor I will use the GPS (don't be stupid!). Other than that I just enjoy the ride. Sometimes I see areas of town that are new to me. Life isn't a race. It is a journey.

The Scariest Blackness

Problem:

The absolute scariest Blackness is when I can't recall events. What happened this morning or yesterday. Or a minute ago.

It can be a small event and time frame or something much larger.

To help a friend I made a trip which involved a flight, an overnight hotel stay, a meeting with some people and a flight home. The next day I started shaking and crying because I knew I had traveled but couldn't recall getting home or anything else about the day before except being in the hotel courtyard in the morning. Blackness. Nothing of the meeting. No idea of the company name. Or how many people we met. Just a huge amount of Blackness. I often try to recall that day just to test myself. As I type this all I get from that day is Blackness. I know I have successfully recalled that event. But most of the time I get Blackness.

I can watch a movie and not be able to recall the movie when it is done (and yes I stayed awake!). Just Blackness.

And once I have problems recalling an event that event is likely to be problematic forever.

Sometimes I come out of the Blackness and can't recall what it was I was trying to remember in the first place. A vicious cycle.

Cope:

First, I now understand what is happening. And I know the Blackness for what it is. This helps reduce the fear.

And instead of trying to recall the information I will ask for help.

Normally the item I failed on is a proper name. The name of a person, city, place or restaurant.

But I can give a description to help someone else come up with the name.

- Hey you remember my high school buddy that bowls? Well, he wants to play cards this weekend.

- Let's go eat at that BBQ place by the mall.

- Your youngest brother called for you.

- I'm going to golf at the course west of town.

- Remember the movie we saw last night?

I also avoid using proper nouns.

- I say "Hey guy" instead of "Hey Steve".

- I say "Call your younger brother" instead of "Call Gord".

- I say "Are you having lunch with the babysitter?" instead of "Are you having lunch with Linda?"

Small changes that decrease the chance of falling into Blackness.

Lots of small successes!

Stress

Problem:

One of the biggest issues I have to deal with is Stress.

I used to thrive on this at work. Loved solving problems. Liked to be a cowboy to solve problems. Dealt with a lot of client issues and programing problems.

Now stress is the number one thing that seems to escalate my problems. Worry. Fretting. Expectations. People watching me. Talking in groups. Timelines.

And of course experiencing a problem creates stress which can make the problem worse. I think this is one of the reasons the problems Compound.

Cope:

Anything I can do to avoid or reduce stress is key. Putting things in perspective.

Time line doesn't matter. Nobody gets hurt.

Everyone has problems. Don't feel bad when people watch me when I have problems.

Exercise. Walking.

Keeping busy.

Feeling like I accomplished something.

Tired

Problem:

I get exhausted easily. Mostly mentally and emotionally but also physically.

During a day when my problems compound I am wiped out. The day might start out fine then cognitive problems start. Then vision. Then headaches.

The back of my head, shoulders and neck can just be tight with pain. After a couple hours of this escalation I am tired.

Vision and cognitive problems will just make me mentally exhausted. Don't want to see anything. Don't want to try to talk. Just want to withdraw.

Cope:

Redefined my expectations of how I will feel. Exhaustion is not bad or failure. It is an everyday occurrence. It is something to conquer.

Take breaks. Use exercise to fight exhaustion. Walk. Lift weights. Do push-ups. Get the blood flowing. Shift the focus if only for ten minutes. Or go for an hour.

Our home walls are mostly blank which helps with sensory overload. However, my cave is a quiet room in the basement where the walls are covered with movie posters, a wall is lined with my remaining books, golf flags, pictures etc. Sometimes my break will be to go in the cave and wander around reliving events. Maybe pull a book off of the shelf and just feel it. Or stand in front of a poster from Comic Con. Instead of taking a break from everything I am focusing on an item or a specific happy memory. Sometimes I go into my office, which has a dozen family pictures. I will focus on one of the pictures of our wedding, kids, grandparents, grandkids etc. Just taking a break with a happy memory.

Naps are only for extreme cases. Maybe a couple times a month when nothing else works. Don't want to sleep my life away.

Sleep

Problem:

After the TBI, I had increased trouble sleeping. Was thinking Bad Thoughts before sleep. Was too exhausted to sleep. Kept replaying the problems of the day. Failures. How could I face them the next day? Headaches made it difficult to sleep. As my headaches escalated my shoulders and neck hurt. Pain in my knee.

Sleep had never been my friend. Most of my life I slept relatively little. Didn't need eight hours. Six hours was a long time for me.

Cope:

My neuropsych helped me significantly with getting to sleep. We went through my habits of trying to sleep. I did the normal things like counting or thinking good thoughts. I would also do weird things like math problems and math drills, or from memory review books or memories that I liked, or reviewing old programs that I had written.

Dr A told me to try putting on a helmet when I was ready to sleep. Not a real helmet but an imaginary helmet. A helmet that didn't allow new thoughts to start and stopped current thought processes. Sounds goofy but I worked at it. And it definitely works...at least for me.

He also told me that getting to sleep works better once you are at peace with yourself. This was a constant theme. Acceptance brings Peace. Peace is foundational for many things in life. Happiness. Sleep.

Slow

Problem:

I am much slower than I used to be when speaking. I also speak less often. This has become normal for me...part of redefining myself. I need to speak slower to do my best to recall the items before I try to speak. However, I now get interrupted constantly. Or people try to fill in the pauses when I speak.

If I am in a high sensory overload setting (more triggers) like a restaurant, bar or office this increases the odds that I will have cognitive problems and speak even slower.

Cope:

My initial reaction was to withdraw. Just avoid talking. That became my default.

Now I try to speak less and speak slower. But increase likelihood of success.

I battle constant interruptions but I expect it and try to keep pushing on at my own speed.

It is definitely a tradeoff. Success at speaking but increased frustration due to people helping or interrupting me.

Understand and Accept.

Knocking Glasses Over

Problem:

If I try to pick up a glass with my left hand I sometimes knock it over.

The eye doctors found that I have a mid-line shift in my vision. Basically what I see as the center of my vision is actually shifted to the right. The vision therapy helped retrain my brain so the problem isn't as pronounced as it initially was after the accident but it still occurs.

Also when my brain isn't processing my left eye input correctly I have problems.

Avoid/Cope:

I have retrained myself to always use my right hand to pick up glasses.

I set them on the right-hand side of my spot at the table to minimize the influence of my left eye.

I will also sometimes eat with my left eye closed if my problems have already escalated.

Rectangles

Problem:

My brain for some stupid reason (as if I understand any of these problems!) now likes to have my eyes trace the outline of rectangles. Not circles or triangles just rectangles!

This following the outlines of rectangles seems to take priority by my brain. Sometimes it gets so severe that my whole body locks up and I just sit or stand and stare. Very weird and scary.

Examples:

Sitting in a restaurant and there are many pictures on the wall opposite me. In one place they had a dozen little windows cut into an interior wall. I completely zoned out. Missed out on conversations, companions and waitresses. Still can't recall those meals.

The store Target is full of rectangles. The floor and ceiling tiles are rectangles and for some reason very noticeable to me. Many times I have taken several steps into Target and just locked up. I stay standing there until something or someone breaks the loop my brain is in.

Another example: the cereal box aisle in the grocery store. Several times I have locked up staring at the cereal boxes. Once this older man was tapping me on the shoulder with his cane when I was locked staring at cereal. I think he was afraid to get closer to me. He kept asking if I was alright. He thought I was having a stroke or that I was stoned. Not sure how long I was there. He said he had watched me for minutes.

Or in meeting rooms where they have plaques and pictures on the walls.

Rectangles are all over. Books in a store. Windows. Frames. Tiles. A few don't cause me problems. But many are trouble.

Cope:

This one is really tough, especially when taken by surprise. When it happens I focus on just laughing it off. These episodes are really embarrassing as they are very noticeable to the people around me.

I always glance at the walls before I choose where to sit in a restaurant. I once walked into a restaurant and the floor and walls were all tiles. And the tables were topped with tiles too. I just turned around and walked out.

In stores I normally take a shopping cart and focus on the handle of the cart as I walk through the store.

If I don't have a cart I look at the back of the person walking in front of me. Or if there aren't many people in the store I look down as much as possible and watch the tips of my shoes. If I have a list I focus on the list.

Reading

Problem:

Reading is very difficult.

Between my memory and vision problems, reading has become very difficult, ineffective and sometimes just impossible.

I used to read three to five books a week or several hundred a year. Reading was a joy. I loved books. The feel of a book. Learning new things. Finding new heroes. Experiencing vicariously. The turn of a great phrase. I had a couple thousand books. When I didn't have a book and was bored I would go back and just review great books from memory.

Reading uses a ton of memory. I never realized how much. The meaning of a word. The words before and after. The sentence before. The paragraphs before. The book before. Prior books in a series. Settings. Characters. It goes on and on. For me this became a minefield of potential failures. Lots of falling into Blackness. Went from being a joy to failure and a generator of Bad Thoughts.

Of course, reading also uses vision. Often I can't see the images on the page clear enough to read.

Avoid/Cope:

This is a classic case of needing to redefine. I have switched to scanning instead of reading every word, every sentence and every paragraph. So reading now is scanning. Different expectations. Not a deep understanding. Not a joy of the word or phrase. Redefined to get a higher-level view of the story or maybe a scene.

Also I don't attempt to read many new books. Much more effective to just scan older books. Reactivate memories. Not new material. So instead of reading three to five books a week I scan that number in a year. More like meeting old friends.

Instead of reading a book in a couple hours now it takes me days or weeks or months to scan it. A couple pages then take a break. Don't stress the brain. Don't Trigger a headache. New definition of success.

I used to have thousands of books. Lots of old friends. I have given away many of them to family and friends. Introduced others to series and authors they haven't had the joy to find. Instead of boxing up the books and donating them to a library I have made it a personal experience. No hurry. Just sharing when the time is right.

Prism

Problem:

Seeing prisms.

I have worn eyeglasses almost my entire life. Now I see a prism when light hits the top of the lens. It has to do with my eyes not being in synch. It is really distracting. Also, it is a trigger for headaches.

Cope:

I found that if I wear a ball cap, the brim of the hat stops light from hitting the top of the lens so no prisms! So I wear a ball cap all the time now.

Sometimes I can tell people are irritated that I have the hat on...at dinner and inside their house. I am sorry it irritates them but it makes me see better and reduces the chance and magnitude of headaches.

Eyes Wide Shut - Interference

Problem:

The more sensory input I get the more likely cognitive problems will surface.

I was working with my eye doctor reading charts with various prism glasses. My head just wasn't working well. I was having trouble saying the name of the letters on the chart. We took a short break. All of a sudden I was saying all of the letters quickly and easily. The doctor was shocked. We did it a couple more times. Same results. Then he said, "Your eyes are shut." We figured out that I had memorized the chart. I couldn't read it with my eyes open but I could recall it from memory fine with my eyes shut! True but weird. So we then experimented with levels of sensory input. Highly susceptible to vision overload. Much harder to read from a chart in a busy room than from a blank wall. Put a chart next to a window and I did worse. Moving items in the background or periphery caused even more problems. Items on my left caused more problems than moving items on my right. He played music from his iPhone. Sound input affected me some but less than vision input.

The doctor experimented with putting strips of tape on my glasses to minimize visual input. It helped some but looked like I was wearing lizard glasses.

Cope:

Sometimes when I am having cognitive problems I try closing my eyes. It helps sometimes. Of course, I don't do this when I am driving or walking!

I try to sit with my back to the room in restaurants.

Wearing a hat with a brim helps to limit what I see. Just that small decrease in the scope of vision can help. The doctor also said that having a constant item like the brim of my hat in my vision helps 'ground' my vision process.

Left Side and Breaks

Problem:

Often my brain does not coordinate the processing of signals from both of my eyes correctly. It is very tiring when this happens. This often happens while watching movies. Or in a room with lots of people. Lots of activity. Long duration.

Cope:

My favorite spot to sit is always on the left side of a theater, restaurant, table, etc. This helps me in several ways. If my brain isn't processing signals correctly from my left eye then it is much easier for me to see what is happening using just my right eye. Also shifting most of the workload to my right eye seems to help balance out the ongoing conflict between my eyes so I tend to avoid a potential headache trigger.

I take breaks. I try to take a break every fifteen minutes or so. Just close my eyes for a minute. Or if I am having problems I will get up to 'go to the bathroom' but I really just get out of the theater or gathering. Get out of the visual overload and noise. Take a break.

Golf

Problem:

After decades of hard work I had got my golf handicap to be in the single digits. In the last year I had improved from a 14 or 15 to a 6. Thrilled. Success. Golf had been my sport and hobby for forty years. Now I was shooting in the 70's or low 80's on a regular basis.

Then after the accident my whole game had changed. And not for the better.

My vision problems plagued me. Sometimes when I start my swing I see two golf balls or the ball moves towards and away from me. When I have problems I actually miss the ball! Or the ball just hits the end of the head of the club. Not good. I tried wearing an eye patch to eliminate the conflict between my two eyes. It helped some but I would lose my distance vision and get headaches. The problems might only be for a single shot or last for three or four holes. I was now shooting +100 or an 80. Just depends on the day. Failures.

The vision problems also effected my putting. The movement of the putter to start the small back swing can mess up my vision. Might miss the ball. Or take a divot on the green. Or completely miss hit. Failures.

And I can't reliably keep score. Lots of 3's and 7's (honestly more 7's than 3's!!!) So I don't use a score card any more. Also had a couple occasions where people accused me of not remembering my score on a hole on purpose. Not a fun experience. I wasn't cheating.

Cope:

Redefine for the focus to be on the experience rather than the score.

Had a series of breakthroughs on the vision issues after lots of trial and error.

I started waggling the club head above the ball. For some reason this series of small movements reduces the occurrences of seeing two golf balls or the ball moving. Somehow it gets my brain used to movement so the swing of the club doesn't trigger problems as often.

I also changed my putting stroke so I look at the hole rather than the ball when I putt. No more vision problems while putting.

I just had to redefine my expectations. Now I just enjoy the good shots. The shanks and the misses just get laughed off.

If I am playing with others and they want to keep score then I ask them to do it. I also let them know that I might need them to help add up the shots per hole. If I get it wrong I am not trying to cheat.

Walking instead of riding gives me exercise and slows me down which is good. Gives me a break. Time to enjoy the sights. Good thoughts. Sometimes I just shut my eyes and enjoy the sun.

Ear Ringing

Problem:

Medication caused constant ringing in my right ear.

My doctor had me try some medication to try to reduce my headaches. He had occasionally had good luck with this medication for over ten years with other patients. It was about the fourth medicine we had tried. With most of these medications you start out on a low dose and ramp it up. After my second week on this medication my right ear started ringing. And ringing. And ringing.

It is now constant. The tone changes but it always rings.

My doctor researched the medicine for a history of causing tinnitus (ringing in the ear). It occurs in 4% of the people that use it. Four percent.

I weaned off the medicine over a couple weeks. The ear ringing persisted.

It is now chronic. Forever.

Avoid/Cope:

The only thing that seems to help is playing music or having some background noise. Nothing else seems to work. Understand. Accept. Live Gracefully.

Weather

Problem:

Weather plays a key role as a Trigger to my problems. We live in Nebraska which seems to have a lot of weather that Triggers escalation of my problems.

Three things about the weather have an effect on my pain levels and cognitive problems:

- Cold. Cold can Trigger instant headaches. My left temple will start to hurt then followed by pain in the back of my head. If I am already experiencing these problems cold will intensify the pain. Cold also makes my compartment(?) scar, left knee and right hip hurt.

- Dampness. Dampness makes my leg and hip hurt. And then pain in my leg and hip can act as a Trigger for my headaches.

- Quick, significant swings in the weather or pressure changes. My knee doctor said I will be a walking barometer and he was right. I can definitely feel pressure changes through pain and stiffness. Also, the swings in weather Trigger my headaches.

Cope:

Not much anyone can do to change the weather. We have discussed moving to an area with a better climate to avoid the cold, damp and weather swings but we have kids and grandkids in Nebraska and have decided to stay put.

I make sure to wear a hat to protect my head as much as possible.

We travel more in the cold months to better climates. We have spent January in Florida or Palm Desert for the last two years. We don't like being away from family but it really helps my head.

85

GRACEFULLY DIMINISHED: LIVING WITH A TRAUMATIC
BRAIN INJURY

Alcohol

Problem:

Sometimes just a single sip of alcohol can Trigger an instant headache. The headache is only at the back of my head. It completely bypasses my normal headache pattern of temple hurting first then back of head. This is the only time that my normal headache pattern is skipped.

Other times I can have multiple drinks and it never acts as a Trigger.

Research on this subject revealed that this is a known issue with people with TBIs. Not every TBI victim has this problem but some do. The articles said research hasn't found any reason for this but many people report just a single drink will Trigger an intense often debilitating pain at the back, bottom of the head.

Red wine seems to be the strongest Trigger followed by dark beers. Mixed drinks seem to be the least likely to cause problems.

Cope:

Obviously this is easy to avoid by just not drinking. So, I often skip drinking, especially when I am already having problems and don't want to Compound the problems. Or if I am in a situation where I need to concentrate like playing cards or games and don't want to risk the cognitive problems.

But sometimes I just love tasting new micro brews. Or I just want a cold one with friends. Or go to a wine tasting. Then I take the chance and sometimes pay the price. Part of it is not letting the TBI completely change my life.

Dominos

Problem:

Pain in other areas of my body often Trigger headaches or cognitive problems.

The body's reaction to pain is often to tense up.

When my knee starts to hurt I know I am risk of a headache. And the headache can cause more cognitive problems.

I think of it as a row of dominos. Knock one over and the rest start to fall too.

Cope:

I try to remove a domino so more can't get knocked over.

When my knee or hip start to hurt I treat this as an early warning. I do what I can to relieve the pain so it doesn't Trigger something else.

I take a really hot shower. Or go for a walk. Or get outside.

Focus on stopping the next domino from falling. Success.

Unwell - NOT

Problem:

When people notice I have problems or even rarer when I tell them, often they reply with something like "sorry give me a call in a couple days when you are over it." Or "have you been to the doctor?"

Even very smart people with experience with these kinds of issues often don't understand. This is my life. Every day. Chronic is forever.

I sometimes try to explain what Chronic really means and the time lines of the plateaus of TBI recovery. And Triggers. And Compounding.

Even when I take the time and emotional energy to try to explain people normally don't get it. They don't see something physically wrong. So they relate it to having a cold. Take two pills and drink a lot of water.

Or they say "don't lose hope." Or "you will be in my prayers."

Hope and prayers are the last thing I want. Instead, if I take the time to explain I really want their Understanding and Acceptance. No sympathy. No Hope. No Prayers. Accept the new me.

Cope:

The main coping on this is simple: Understand that other people are outside of your control.

Maybe find some new friends.

Stay focused on what you can change. Understand. Accept. Live Gracefully.

If I Want Help...

Problem:

People, once they know I have problems (and I am pretty good at hiding it for just this reason), tend to start doing things for me. Guessing what I can't remember. Speaking for me when I am speaking slow. Giving directions when I can't recall the route or destination. On and on.

I know people are just being nice but it is highly frustrating and demeaning. I can still do things so let me do it even if it might take longer. Life isn't a race. It is a journey. I will get there eventually.

And they get offended when I say I can do it on my own!

Cope:

No good solutions.

Most of the time I just keep my mouth shut. This is one of the problems that still makes me feel like a failure. If the person keeps doing it I will politely try to tell them: Thank you but if I want help I will ask!

Other People

Problem:

I can only change what I do. I can't change others.

Many times I tried unsuccessfully to change how others treat me.

People will talk slower and louder to me after they find out I have a TBI.

They say something and then explain it to me.

Or they give me instructions on how to do simple things.

Cope:

I thought of having a shirt made that said, "Memory Problems. Not Stupid".

A little bit of knowledge is dangerous. Sometimes I will take the time to explain in detail what I can and can't do...and that sometimes helps how I get treated but not always.

Finally it reaches a point where I have to Understand and Accept that each person will treat me differently.

Sometimes it will be very helpful and I can feel successful.

Other times it will be unintentionally demeaning and frustrating.

Just have to roll with it and move on.

Friends

Problem:

You will lose friends.

Several doctors warned me of this. I figured nah won't happen to me.

This was incredibly hard for me. I had always been lucky and had many friends. I still had my core group of high school friends even after thirty years. Most of my friends came from work. I had worked there for over 25 years. Many, many good friends. We did a bunch of things together.

Now that my problems have forced me to quit working I have lost most of those friends. We have just moved on. Sad to miss seeing them.

Cope:

I have gained a very close group of friends. As I started to replace activities that now result in failures with things I can now do a group of work acquaintances have become very good friends. They understand my problems. They aren't put off by them. They don't offer to help unless I ask (which is a miracle). For example, we get together once a month to play games (typically board or strategy games). Reading the rules just doesn't work for me any more so one or two of the guys just do that by default now. They know I can't and I have asked them to do it. No embarrassment. No failure.

One of my favorite games (Smash Up - highly recommended!) involves some simple math. The players need to add up a short string of single digit numbers such as 1+3+3+4. Some nights I can't do it. Other nights I can. On the nights I can I do it my friends don't help. Other nights when I have trouble I ask for help and they just help. Perfect.

Also gained another group of friends that we vacation and play golf together. They also know of my problems. They help when I ask - otherwise they don't. They have also gotten very good about not interrupting me. Perfect again.

And then there are my high school buddies. No problem there. When I ask they help otherwise they leave me alone. They understand my issues and that I have changed. They occasionally ask to understand. They have accepted and supported the new me.

Understand. Accept. Live Gracefully.

However, I have lost other groups of friends.

A large group were work acquaintances. Since I don't work we just don't see each other much. Understandable. Probably typical of when someone retires (voluntarily or otherwise). But still seemed like a failure.

And there is another group of work friends. Some lost interest in me when I couldn't help their careers. Maybe we weren't such good friends.

And we had a group of friends that came over about once a month for wine parties. We stopped having parties because groups are harder for me to handle (more interference and sensory overload.) Now we just have another couple or two over.

Then there was a group of friends that never adjusted to the new me. I tried explaining. They never understood and accepted. Always talking about trivia, books, movies, things we did at work, sports etc. I kept failing. They kept asking what was wrong with me. I guess I didn't act handicapped enough for them to understand and accept me. It got depressing to be around them. They were obviously uncomfortable with me. So we mutually drifted apart.

Coping with losing friends was tough but I had to find peace with it or hop on the emotional roller coaster. Time helps. Finding new friends help. Understanding myself more helps. Knowing friends drift apart normally but that my TBI problems accelerated it. It probably would have happened to some degree anyway.

Kids Don't Judge

Problem:

We spend a lot of time with our grandkids. They are very perceptive when something starts to go wrong.

I was in the basement with four of them (ages 8-11). We were just goofing around. I started to talk to one of them and couldn't recall his name. I locked up for a couple seconds. All of the kids noticed. They thought I was pretending. They all started insisting that I had to say their names. Normally I avoided their names as much as possible to avoid exactly this problem. Pretty soon I was completely locked up. Couldn't recall any of their names. The kids started to realize that something was very wrong. They got very quiet. Two of them hugged me. I had to get up and escape to the bathroom.

I was at the grocery store with our 11-year-old grandson. I was staring at an area of the shelves for what must have been a very long time. My grandson asked what I was looking for. When I told him he pointed right in front of me and laughed. We moved on to a different area. The second time this happened he didn't laugh. He just held my hand and helped me find the item. The third time he took the list and said he could do it.

We were working on math. I have found the best way to help the kids is to make learning fun. Well, our grandson thought I was goofing when I locked up checking his work. He laughed. Then he noticed tears running down my face. He just patted my hand and said it would be okay.

Cope:

After each of these events I had a talk with the kids to explain what had happened and that it was from me getting hit by the bus. We had some long talks. Especially with two of the grandkids. They were interested but very concerned. One of them asked why I wasn't sad. I said the small things didn't matter. I understood and accepted who I was. That everyone has issues to deal with. Some of mine were from getting my head hit. We talked about the math problems I have. I can still help guide the kids on how to add or multiply even if sometimes I can't get the answer myself.

Those discussions were very hard.

The funny thing is the kids just accepted who I was much better than the adults. No judging.

Shame

Problem:

One of the reoccurring issues I deal with is Shame.

Shame is one of the issues that happens when I am not at Peace.

Ashamed I can't earn money.

Ashamed I knocked over a glass at a restaurant.

Ashamed I have to ask someone to total my credit card receipt.

Ashamed I can't sign my name.

Ashamed I don't know my address.

Shame accelerates the downward spirals.

Cope:

I try to put things in perspective.

Nobody was hurt because I didn't know my address...and I was able to retrieve it off of my driver's license.

Probably nobody laughed.

I already knew it was a problem.

No surprise. Just deal with it and move on.

Multiple times a day I review my accomplishments.

Maybe I helped a grandkid. Or had a nice walk. Or made someone laugh. Or caught a fish.

When I start in on a downward spiral I use those accomplishments to stop the spiral and lift me back up.

Emotional - Tears

Problem:

Since the TBI my emotions are just raw. Bad emotions. Good emotions.

I tear up a lot.

When watching a movie or show I get emotional. It doesn't have to be a tear jerker movie just intense. The better I like the movie the more emotional I get.

Cope:

This is one where I can't do much except understand and accept. I can't avoid the situations. A lot of times the triggers are good situations.

Again, I step out from the TV show or movie and give myself a break.

What I can do is to not be embarrassed or feel terrible.

Emotional - Doubt

Problem:

So many failures had filled me with constant doubt. Doubt eats at a person. It changes who you are.

I stopped doing things because of self-doubt. Led to a lot of Bad Thoughts.

Cope:

Define activities to increase chances of success.

I don't put a timer on what I need to do. Just celebrate getting it done. Some days are more difficult. Maybe my vision starts to go bad and I need to pull over and walk for twenty minutes. Maybe I can't recall the route or where I am going so I take the long way. Maybe I forget completely where I am going and have to start over. Life isn't a race. It is a journey. So sometimes I unintentionally take the path less chosen.

Celebrate each accomplishment.

My wife now pays most of our bills. I retained paying our health insurance. Wasn't ready to give up everything. Still prove to myself that I can do it. It is scheduled on my electronic calendar. Some days it takes me several attempts to get it done correctly. Sometimes the subtraction in the checkbook is difficult and I make a mistake. I always check my work. I write down our return address instead of using the little stickers. A couple times I had to look at my driver's license to get our address correct. It is not uncommon for me to be sweating as I do it. But the important thing is that I always get it done on the scheduled date. Got it done! And I celebrate.

Going to stores is a minefield of Triggers. I try to go at least once a day. Maybe to get groceries. Or something for the grandkids. Or just to walk around. I practice my coping techniques. Some days I come out with a killer headache. But I go and do it. And feel good that I did it.

I love driving. Sometimes I will just pick a location and drive to it. Might end up taking a long route but I get there and turn around and drive somewhere else. Maybe home. Maybe to the golf course. But I do it and feel good.

Today I stood in front of some shelves at a pharmacy looking for contact cleaning solution. Cheated - had a picture of the old bottle on my phone! Must have tried ten times to find the item my wife wanted. Walked away several times. Still couldn't see the right box. Saw a lot of boxes but the names and images just weren't making sense. Finally walked away and came back with my left eye closed. Found it right away. Weird huh? Didn't get frustrated. Knew I had all of the time I needed to find it. Just kept trying different ways until my brain clicked. Got it done. Success.

Errands aren't chores...they are opportunities to be successful.

The only thing that fights doubt is success. Might be a small success but still a success. Many small successes add up.

Withdrawal

Problem:

I started to withdraw from everything.

Friends

Events

Activities

Going out in public

Golfing

Everything

It was a very normal reaction but very, very dangerous. Doctors had warned me about withdrawing.

Without things to fill time there was a lot of time for Bad Thoughts. It became a bad cycle.

Cope:

I had to redefine who I was and what I wanted to do. And part of that new definition had to involve people.

Also I had to Understand and Accept that with interactions came pain, embarrassment, frustrations and sometimes Bad Thoughts. But that level of negatives was much better than where the constant withdrawal would lead. I had to break the cycle in small steps. Go to the store. Go with a group. Walk among people and notice they don't point and stare. Golf but don't worry about keeping score. Small changes.

I go to Comic Con. Tens of thousands of people. When it gets to be more than I can handle I go sit on the steps and look at the harbor. Or walk around the docks. Just take a break. Maybe ten or more breaks a day. But I go. I go with a handful of good friends. They know I set my own schedule and activities. No pressure. It is fun. And it is a personal challenge. And I am successful.

Games

Problem:

My cognitive and vision problems stopped me from playing many of the games that were my hobby.

I had always been a Gamer from a very young age. My brother and I played thousands of hours on Avalon Hill, Monopoly, pinball, video and other types of games. More recently I had played hundreds of hours of games on the PC such as Civilization. I loved strategy type games.

My grandkids loved to play Xbox games with me like football and basketball. Vision problems make it very frustrating to play games that included many moving pieces. The movement triggers vision problems such as double vision and shifting vision. Also headaches can be triggered. Plus I wasn't able to be effective at the games any more. Failures instead of fun.

Games such as Civilization included many small icons and a large board. I had played Civilization for years for thousands of hours. Both my vision and recall problems stopped me from playing games like this. Very frustrating. Triggered headaches and vision problems. Failures.

Cope:

I had to shift to simpler games that involved much less movement and detail and that didn't require much memory recall. I kept trying to go back to old favorites but way too many triggers. Also had to find games that I could play by myself so when I had problems I could just stop playing without feeling peer pressure to continue.

So I searched and found games that I can still play. It took a lot of searching. But it worked.

Sometimes I still play games that will Trigger headaches but I do it knowing the risk. Yes, this game Triggered problems before but my friends want to play it. So I choose to play it to be with my friends.

A very good example of Understanding and Accepting. Then changing and redefining to fit with what I could be successful at. Basically learning that I didn't have to give up hobbies I just had to figure out how to live gracefully.

Cheats

Cheats in video games are a way of playing, moving or entering a code to gain an advantage. I seldom used them as I preferred to play without the advantage.

Now with dealing the TBI problems I decided to find as many Life Cheats as possible.

There are scores of ways I have found to use technology to help or mask my problems. Also technology has gotten to the point where the information is backed up many ways.

1. Pictures

If I am having a bad day and the guys are coming over to play board games I will make a list of who is coming over. Or once they are at the house I draw the table on a piece of paper with their names where they are sitting. I then take a picture of the seating map using my phone. I could have just used the paper but that can draw attention to my problem and make me less likely to use the aid. By having the picture on my phone I can reference as needed. People will think I am checking email or Facebook instead of seeing what their names are.

I also use pictures to keep track of important information. Medications. My address. Birthdays.

When traveling I take pictures of our rental car, where it is parked, our hotel room number etc. This trick is wonderful. No stress of having to remember changing information. I just look at a picture on my phone.

Pictures are also easy to delete once you don't need the information on the note.

2. TripAdvisor

Not only does it help pick out places to eat or stay it has become my memory on where we did things and how we liked it. Removes a lot of the pressure. And it is fun writing down the reviews. If I am having problems I can wait to write the review when I am functioning better.

3. Notes

I make notes in my phone of simple things. Names of restaurants. A city. A golf course. Lots of things throughout the day. And then I clean up the notes when I don't need the info any more.

4. Calendar

Lots of time I don't know what the day of the week is...or the date. Or sometimes the month. Oddly I do a good job of remembering when to do things or to meet people...just often don't remember where! My phone's calendar solves most of these issues. And people don't think it is weird.

5. GPS/Mapquest

Often I forget how to get home. Or the route to somewhere I have just been or have been many times. My car's GPS is awesome.

6. Facebook

Social media is good in moderation. Most of the sentences or posts are short. I can process them more successfully than a long email. And I can respond or post based upon my own schedule - when I am cognitively functioning at a high level. The ability to schedule based off of my current ability level is terrific.

7. DVR/Video Streaming

This has been a lifesaver. I might have had to give up watching TV and movies completely. Now we record the shows we want to watch and play them when we want. We can fast forward through the dreaded commercials! Most importantly I can schedule when we watch based upon the unpredictability of how I am feeling. We can pause the shows and I can take breaks while watching a show...get up and walk around, let the dog outside, just close my eyes and shut everything out.

Tradeoffs

With all of these examples and dozens of other situations there are always tradeoffs.

As Newton said, "For each action there is an equal and opposite reaction."

No perfect solution.

Each decision has an opposite reaction:

- Walking may make headaches better but my knee hurts.

- Music helps mask the ringing in my ear but can Trigger sensory overload.

- Wearing a hat helps but it peeves people off.

- Taking on an activity can bring success but it often Triggers a headache or vision problem.

Understanding makes each of these a thoughtful decision on the path to living Gracefully Diminished.

PART SEVEN
That's All Folks

Hope this helps someone!

Good Luck

1.7 million people experience a Traumatic Brain Injury every year (Source: CDC). You are not alone.

If you think you have a TBI go to a doctor right away. The brain recovers in plateaus over the first nine to twelve months. Some TBIs are not obvious. Get help quickly to help the brain help itself.

A Traumatic Brain Injury is forever. The problems it creates vary by person. No two people are affected the same. The problems don't have to make sense. You will be Diminished. But you can still be successful. Redefine yourself for success.

Don't rely on Hope. Hope is a downhill emotional roller coaster.

Work on Understanding, then Acceptance, then Living Gracefully.

The wisdom and courage to Understand and make changes.

The process never ends. It is ongoing.

Hopefully this has helped you in some way.

Maybe you recognized a similar problem.

Maybe you found a path or don't feel so alone.

Maybe you found something you can relate to and will feel better and stay away from Bad Thoughts.

Understand. Accept. Live Gracefully.

To paraphrase the Most Interesting Man in the World: 'Stay Graceful My Friends.'